OBESITY AND OVERWEIGHT: ALL YOU NEED TO KNOW ABOUT OBESITY AND OVERWEIGHT AND ITS PREVENTION

BY

Dr. Jennifer Godwin

Copyright@2022Dr.JenniferGodwin

TABLE OF CONTENTS

INTRODUCTION

Chapter one

Facts about overweight and obesity

Chapter two

What causes overweight and obesity

Chapter three

Ways to regulate body fats and prevent overweight and obesity

Conclusion

INTRODUCTION

OVERWEIGHT AND OBESITY

Overweight and obesity are characterized as strange or unreasonable fat amassing that might impede wellbeing.

Weight list (BMI) is a basic file of weight-for-level that is regularly used to characterize overweight and obesity in grown-ups. It is characterized as an individual's load in kilograms separated by the square of his level in meters (kg/m2).

ADULTS

For Adults, WHO characterizes overweight and obesity as follows:

overweight is a BMI more noteworthy than or equivalent to 25; and Obesity is a BMI more prominent than or equivalent to 30.

BMI gives the most helpful populace level proportion of overweight and obesity as it is no different for the two genders and for all times of grown-ups. In any case, it ought to be viewed as an unpleasant aide since it may not relate in a similar way of obesity in various people.

CHAPTER ONE

FACTS ABOUT OVERWEIGHT AND OBESITY

Some new WHO worldwide appraisals follow.

In 2016, more than 1.9 billion grown-ups matured 18 years and more seasoned were overweight. Of these more than 650 million grown-ups were large.

In 2016, 39% of grown-ups matured 18 years and more than (39% of men and 40% of ladies) were overweight.

Generally speaking, around 13% of the world's grown-up populace (11% of men and 15% of ladies) were corpulent in 2016.

The overall pervasiveness of obesity almost significantly increased somewhere in the range of 1975 and 2016.

In 2019, an expected 38.2 million kids younger than 5 years were overweight or obesity. When considered a major league salary country issue, overweight and corpulence are currently on the ascent in low-and center pay nations, especially in metropolitan settings. In Africa, the quantity of overweight youngsters under 5 has expanded by almost 24% percent starting around 2000. Close to half of the youngsters under 5 who were overweight or fat in 2019 lived in Asia.

North of 340 million youngsters and teenagers matured 5-19 were overweight or fat in 2016.

The predominance of overweight and obesity among youngsters and teenagers matured 5-19 has risen decisively from only 4% in 1975 to simply more than 18% in 2016. The ascent has happened much the same way among both young men and young ladies: in 2016 18% of young ladies and 19% of young men were overweight.

While just shy of 1% of kids and youths matured 5-19 were hefty in 1975, more 124 million youngsters and teenagers (6% of young ladies and 8% of young men) were corpulent in 2016.

Overweight and underweight are connected to additional passings overall than underweight. All around the world there are a greater number of individuals who are large than underweight - this happens in each locale with the exception of parts of sub-Saharan Africa and Asia.

CHAPTER TWO

WHAT CAUSES OVERWEIGHT AND OBESITY

The principal reason for obesity and overweight is an energy irregularity between calories consumed and calories exhausted. Worldwide, there has been: an expanded admission of energy-thick food sources that are high in fat and sugars; and an expansion in actual dormancy because of the undeniably stationary nature of many types of work, changing methods of transportation, and expanding urbanization.

Changes in dietary and active work designs are much of the time the consequence of natural and cultural changes related with improvement and absence of steady strategies in areas, for example, wellbeing, horticulture, transport, metropolitan preparation, climate, food handling, conveyance, advertising, and training.

Complications of Overweight and Obesity

Raised BMI is a significant gamble factor for noncommunicable sicknesses, for example,

cardiovascular illnesses (for the most part coronary illness and stroke), which were the main source of death in 2012; diabetes;

outer muscle issues (particularly osteoarthritis - a profoundly impairing degenerative sickness of the joints);

a few tumors (counting endometrial, bosom, ovarian, prostate, liver, gallbladder, kidney, and colon).

The gamble for these noncommunicable illnesses increments, with expansions in BMI.

Youth weight is related with a higher opportunity of heftiness, sudden passing and handicap in adulthood. Yet, notwithstanding expanded future dangers, hefty kids experience breathing troubles, expanded hazard of cracks, hypertension, early markers of cardiovascular sickness, insulin obstruction and mental impacts.

CHAPTER THREE

WAYS TO REGULATE BODY FATS AND PREVENT OVERWEIGHT AND OBESITY

Picking better food varieties (entire grains, products of the soil, sound fats and protein sources) and refreshments. Restricting undesirable food sources (refined grains and desserts, potatoes, red meat, handled meat) and refreshments (sweet beverages), Expanding active work

Restricting TV time, screen time, and other "sit time",Further developing rest, Decreasing pressure

10 Methods for preventing overweight and obesity

1: Hydrate

Stoutness is a serious danger to sound way of life. Hence, on World Stoutness Day, we let you know straightforward ways of forestalling this wellbeing danger...

2: water

Drinking more water goes about as hunger suppressant; thus you eat less

3:Take a Walk

A decent stroll for 30 minutes will help your heart and brain.

4:Utilize Less Salt

Utilize less salt in your eating regimen and keep a sound circulatory strain.

5: Exercise

Practice YogaPractise different yoga asans for weight reduction.

6:Eat Green Vegetables

Remember green veggies for your eating regimen, something like one time each week.

7: Eat fruits

Continuously convey apples and oranges to work. Eat natural products when desires for snacks sets in.

8: Keep away from Sugar

Quit eating sweet food, as sugar is the genuine lowlife for spreading the corpulence scourge.

9: Never Skip Breakfast

Avoiding the primary dinner of the day will make you more eager, which will give you cheap food desires.

10: Work out

Require out no less than a little ways from your bustling timetable to work out

CONCLUSION

Weight record (BMI) is an estimation that considers an individual's weight and level to gauge body size.

In grown-ups, obesity is characterized as having a BMI of 30.0
Obesity is related with a higher gamble for serious infections, like sort 2 diabetes, coronary illness, and disease.

Yet, BMI isn't all that matters. It has a few restrictions as a measurement.

"Factors like age, sex, identity, and bulk can impact the connection among BMI and muscle to fat ratio. Likewise, BMI doesn't recognize overabundance fat, muscle, or bone mass, nor does it give any sign of the conveyance of fat among people."

Notwithstanding these constraints, BMI keeps on being broadly utilized as a method for estimating body size.

How is obesity classified?

The accompanying classesTrusted Source are utilized for grown-ups who are something like 20 years of age:

BMI   Class

18.5   underweight

18.5 to <25.0   "normal" weight

25.0 to <30.0   overweight

30.0 to <35.0   class 1 corpulence

35.0 to <40.0   class 2 corpulence

40.0 or over class 3 corpulence (otherwise called horrible, outrageous, or serious heftiness)

What is adolescence corpulence?

For a specialist to analyze a kid more than 2 years of age or a youngster with stoutness, their BMI must be in the 95th percentileTrusted Source for individuals of their equivalent age and natural sex:

Percentile scope of BMI Class

>5% underweight

5% to <85% "normal" weight

85% to <95% overweight

95% or obesity

From 2015 to 2016, 18.5 percentTrusted Source (or around 13.7 million) American youth somewhere in the range of 2 and 19 years of age were considered to have clinical stoutness.

What causes weight?

Eating a bigger number of calories than you consume in everyday action and exercise — on a drawn out premise — can prompt corpulence. Over the long haul, these additional calories add up and cause weight gain.

Yet, it's not generally pretty much calories in and calories out, or having a stationary way of life. While those are without a doubt reasons for corpulence, certain purposes you have no control over.

Normal explicit reasons for corpulence include:

hereditary qualities, which can influence how your body processes food into energy and how fat is put away
becoming older, which can prompt less bulk and a more slow metabolic rate, making it simpler to put on weight
not resting enough, which can prompt hormonal changes that cause you to feel

hungrier and long for specific fatty food varieties

pregnancy, as weight acquired during pregnancy might be hard to lose and could ultimately prompt corpulence

Certain medical issue can likewise prompt weight gain, which might prompt stoutness. These include:

polycystic ovary disorder (PCOS), a condition that causes a lopsidedness of female conceptive chemicals

Prader-Willi disorder, an interesting condition present upon entering the world that causes exorbitant yearning Cushing disorder, a condition brought about by having high cortisol levels (the pressure chemical) in your framework

hypothyroidism (underactive thyroid), a condition where the thyroid organ doesn't create enough of specific significant chemicals

osteoarthritis (OA) and different circumstances that cause torment that might prompt decreased movement

Who is at Risk for Obesity or Overweight ?

A mind boggling blend of variables can build an individual's gamble for heftiness.

1: Hereditary qualities

Certain individuals have qualities that make it hard for them to get more fit.

2: Climate and local area

Your current circumstance at home, at school, and locally can all impact how and what you eat, and how dynamic you are.

You might be at a higher gamble for heftiness on the off chance that you:

live in a neighborhood with restricted good food choices or with manyTrusted Source fatty food choices, similar to drive-through joints haven't yet figured out how to prepare quality dinners

try not to figure you can bear the cost of better food varieties

haven't foundTrusted Source a decent spot to play, walk, or practice in your area

3: Mental and different variables

Sadness can once in a while prompt weight gain, as certain individuals might go to nourishment for close to home solace. Certain antidepressants can likewise expand the gamble of weight gain.

3: Stopping smoking: is dependably something to be thankful for, yet stopping might prompt weight gain as well. In certain individuals, it might prompt excessiveTrusted Source weight gain.

Hence, it's vital to zero in on diet and exercise while you're stopping, to some degree after the underlying withdrawal period.

4:Drugs

Drugs for example, steroids or anti-conception medication pills, can likewise raise your gamble for weight gain.

How is obesity analyzed?

BMI is an unpleasant computation of an individual's load corresponding to their level.

Other more exact proportions of muscle versus fat and muscle to fat ratio dispersion include:

skinfold thickness tests

abdomen to-hip correlations

screening tests, for example, ultrasounds, CT sweeps, and MRI filters. Your primary care physician may likewise arrange specific tests to assist with diagnosing stoutness related wellbeing gambles. These may include:

blood tests to look at cholesterol and glucose levels

liver capability tests

a diabetes screening

thyroid tests

heart tests, like an electrocardiogram (ECG or EKG)

An estimation of the fat around your midriff is likewise a decent indicator of your gamble for weight related illnesses.